Prabhuraj Sabarad
Sonali Rai

Relapse Retention and Retainers in Orthodontics

Amit Prakash
Prabhuraj Sabarad
Sonali Rai

Relapse Retention and Retainers in Orthodontics

LAP LAMBERT Academic Publishing

Impressum / Imprint

Bibliografische Information der Deutschen Nationalbibliothek: Die Deutsche Nationalbibliothek verzeichnet diese Publikation in der Deutschen Nationalbibliografie; detaillierte bibliografische Daten sind im Internet über http://dnb.d-nb.de abrufbar.

Alle in diesem Buch genannten Marken und Produktnamen unterliegen warenzeichen-, marken- oder patentrechtlichem Schutz bzw. sind Warenzeichen oder eingetragene Warenzeichen der jeweiligen Inhaber. Die Wiedergabe von Marken, Produktnamen, Gebrauchsnamen, Handelsnamen, Warenbezeichnungen u.s.w. in diesem Werk berechtigt auch ohne besondere Kennzeichnung nicht zu der Annahme, dass solche Namen im Sinne der Warenzeichen- und Markenschutzgesetzgebung als frei zu betrachten wären und daher von jedermann benutzt werden dürften.

Bibliographic information published by the Deutsche Nationalbibliothek: The Deutsche Nationalbibliothek lists this publication in the Deutsche Nationalbibliografie; detailed bibliographic data are available in the Internet at http://dnb.d-nb.de.

Any brand names and product names mentioned in this book are subject to trademark, brand or patent protection and are trademarks or registered trademarks of their respective holders. The use of brand names, product names, common names, trade names, product descriptions etc. even without a particular marking in this works is in no way to be construed to mean that such names may be regarded as unrestricted in respect of trademark and brand protection legislation and could thus be used by anyone.

Coverbild / Cover image: www.ingimage.com

Verlag / Publisher:
LAP LAMBERT Academic Publishing
ist ein Imprint der / is a trademark of
AV Akademikerverlag GmbH & Co. KG
Heinrich-Böcking-Str. 6-8, 66121 Saarbrücken, Deutschland / Germany
Email: info@lap-publishing.com

Herstellung: siehe letzte Seite /
Printed at: see last page
ISBN: 978-3-659-32882-4

Copyright © 2013 AV Akademikerverlag GmbH & Co. KG
Alle Rechte vorbehalten. / All rights reserved. Saarbrücken 2013

TABLE OF CONTENTS

Introduction

In 1904, Victor Hugo Jackson said, "Not infrequently cases are presented that require more skill in retaining the teeth than in regulating them." Edward A. Angle wrote in 1907, "Retention is too often lightly considered." Both statements may seem quaint or even casual to the orthodontist of the computer age, but these pioneers and others with similar concerns posed the problem of retention or its counterpart— relapse or treatment instability. The problem has not been satisfactorily answered by the multiplicity of authoritative statements and opinions, or by clinical and experimental studies made before and during the intervening decades.

Despite this lack of definiteness of the studies to be reviewed, to achieve some clarity and understanding of the magnitude of the retention problem, it would seem to be not only an advantage but almost a prerequisite for the serious clinical orthodontist and the researcher to be familiar with the approaches and studies that have already been made. In doing so, he or she will better appreciate some of the variation in the treatment results that are being retained and the complex nature of the retention problem.

Moreover, the complexity of the retention problem is very often increased because the clinician, the researcher, and the patient can and do view retention in very different lights with almost endless gradation. For example, the problem will differ if the clinician has to make a choice for a particular patient in obtaining a more desirable facial result at the possible expense of optimal occlusal stability. On the other hand, the academic and more research-oriented orthodontist often gathers statistics and evaluates them without having to become involved with either the esthetic or psychological needs of the patient.

Orthodontic literature has focused to a great extent on the nature of tooth movement and the associated Biomechanics and tissue reactions, However the other side of the problem, the reaction of supporting tissues that becomes manifest at various periods following appliance removal and the nature and extent of the relapse that is almost certain to some degree following orthodontic correction has not been dealt with to the same extent.

In many instances, the most difficult phase of orthodontic treatment is not the active movement of teeth but the retention of the teeth in their new positions. Volumes have been written on causes and prevention of retention failures, but to date the difficulties involved in the retention period of orthodontic therapy have not been eliminated. Additional knowledge of facial growth and development, greatly improved techniques of orthodontic mechanics and the recent advances in diagnosis of the various factors in dentofacial deformities have all enabled the orthodontist to obtain better treatment results – results that would seem less prone to cause problems in the retention phases of treatment. There is, nevertheless, much to be learned about tooth movement, and there is probably even more to be learned concerning maintenance of the teeth after they have been moved.

Biologic nature of dental relapse

Horowitz and Hixon (1969) suggested that Normal physiologic forces beyond the orthodontist's control may result in post treatment occlusion or alignment changes (for example, lower incisor crowding). Biologically, these variations represent a recovery of rebound of the individual's dental development pattern. As the "normal" developmental process was disturbed to an extent by orthodontic interference, then, the post treatment changes rightfully may be considered as recovery, or a physiologic return toward the patient's original condition.

In addition to physiologic recovery, normal growth changes must be included as contributing to the continuous adaptation process that sustains the long term stability of the dental apparatus. Further, since these growth changes are no different in nature and magnitude from those that often occur in untreated persons, there is good reason to differentiate between them and relapse.

They defined the phenomena as follows

Physiologic recovery The type of post treatment changes that represent a rebound or reversion toward the original malocclusion. Examples are rotations, lower anterior crowding, collapse following arch expansion, molar relationship changes, and recurrence of overbite (or open-bite) and overjet.

Developmental changes (both adolescent and adult). The type of post treatment changes that would be anticipated, whether or not orthodontic therapy had intervened. Examples

4

are lower incisor crowding, changes in overbite, and variations in the amount and direction of maxillary and mandibular growth.

Edwards (1968) studied the changes in the periodontium during orthodontic rotation of teeth. Orthodontic appliances were constructed on 6 young experimental dogs to rotate the maxillary second incisors. The attached gingival and to some extent, the mucosa did follow in the direction of rotation. In the free gingival fiber groups of the marginal region, a marked displacement and apparent stretching of the fibrous structures were routinely observed. The transseptal fibers of the rotated teeth also showed a consistent displacement.

He suggested that the fibrous elements of the periodontium adapt to tooth movement in possibly three ways : (1) progressive osteogenic activity (and cementogenic activity to a far lesser degree) plays an active role in the shortening of the extended fibers and in the reattachment of new fibers developed during the tooth movement ; (2) the stretching of the wavy collagen fibers and reorientation of their directional morphology permits a certain amount of tooth movement ; (3) the existence of a type of intermediate plexus might allow an elongation of fiber bundles by "slippage" of the fibers over one another and a subsequent reorientation of the fibers in the new position.

The final return of the slow – metabolizing connective tissue fibers to their original and stable relationship to the tooth and to each other depends on the remodeling of the osseous tissue. The supracrestal fibers, of course, do not have the plastic osseous tissue to eliminate their distortions after tooth movement; thus, they remain in a taut and deviated position for long periods of time.

The fibers of the gingiva remain attached to the tooth during orthodontic rotation, which results in a displacement of the gingiva in the direction of tooth movement.

The transseptal and gingival fibers were still taut and oriented in the direction of rotation thus inducing relapse upon discontinuation of retention.

Reitan (1959) upon studying the nature of relapse found that newly formed bone spicules will be rearranged so as to form a layer of bone containing clefts and future marrow spaces around the capillaries. If the tooth is not retained, it may relapse and cause compression, and occasionally hyalinization, on the former tension side. This is then followed by rearrangement and compression of the more or less calcified bundle bone layer. It is thus important to retain the teeth until fibrous tissue has rearranged and the new bone layers have been calcified.

While the principal fibers of the periodontal ligament rearrange themselves after a period of 8 to 9 weeks, the supra-alveolar structures behave differently and may remain stretched for a longer period. In the supra-alveolar group, formerly called the circular ligament and considered of importance in maintaining the tooth position, there is apparently a slower turnover, as indicated by the scarcity of new cells. This may partly explain why the supra-alveolar fibers rearrange so much later than the principal fibers. Clinical observations have revealed also that these fibers will become relaxed and rearranged after a longer period of time. The difference in reaction between supra-alveolar and principal fibers is of great clinical significance. If a tooth or a group of teeth is released immediately after fairly rapid movement, all the fibers of the periodontal ligament tend to contract and rearrange themselves to their original positions.

Redlich et al (1996) reevaluated the validity of the hitherto assumed causes for the relapse of orthodontic rotations that stretched supraalveolar gingival fibres pulled back the tooth and brought about relaxation of the stretched fibres by obtaining ultra structural data on the response of collagen fibres after orthodontic intervention. Lateral maxillary incisors in the dog were rotated with bonded fixed appliances. The teeth were divided into groups according to different orthodontic procedures. Scanning and transmission electron microscopic analysis were performed on gingival samples after proper processing. Analysis of the untreated control samples showed well-organized, parallel, and densely packed thick bundles of collagen fibres, interconnected with thin fibres. After rotation–followed–by–retention, the gingival fibres were torn, ripped, disorganized, and laterally spaced and of increased diameter. Thus it was concluded that all these patterns are incompatible with stretching. Also, an increased number of elastic fibres were seen in proximity to the torn collagen fibres and it was it was this that contributed to relapse. After gingival fiberotomy, most fibres assumed the appearance of the organized pattern of large fibber bundles similar to those seen in the controls.

Robert Litowitz (1948) in his study indicated that molar teeth, disturbed by orthodontic treatment, have a strong tendency to return toward their original relationships within their respective jaws after treatment. In the case of the mandibular molars it has been shown that these teeth may be moved bodily, or by tipping forces, in either a mesial or distal direction by orthodontic forces. Regardless of the type or direction of movement, however, the majority of cases showed a tendency for this tooth to return to its original position.

Assessment of relapse following orthodontic correction

Dugoni et al (1995)   assessed the long-term stability of mandibular incisors in patients treated in the early mixed dentition by the preservation of leeway space with a passive lingual arch.

Twenty-five patients who underwent early mixed dentition treatment were evaluated during the following stages: pre-treatment (early mixed dentition), phase 2 (early permanent dentition), and postretention (average of 9.5 years). All patients were treated with a removable passive lingual arch. The lingual arch was as effective as fixed edgewise appliances in the reduction of anterior crowding. Intercanine and intermolar widths increased significantly during treatment, and intermolar width was held postretention. Intercanine width decreased significantly during postretention. Mandibular arch length did not decrease during the mixed dentition, but decreased during the postretention stage. The lower incisor alignment was clinically acceptable in 76% of cases in the postretention stage.

Little, Riedel, and Engst (1991)   evaluated long-term serial records of patients who had undergone serial extraction plus comprehensive treatment and retention. All cases were treated with standard edgewise mechanics and were judged clinically satisfactory by the end of active treatment. There was no difference between the serial extraction sample and a matched sample extracted and treated after eruption of a full complement of teeth.

 Arch length and arch width decrease along with increased crowding was similar to orthodontically treated first premolar serial extraction cases. This current evidence continuing to confirm the view that postretention irregularity is an inevitable response in

9

cases with inadequate pre-treatment arch length. Serial extraction cases will likely continue to worsen as they age but with less significant deterioration after age.

Little, Wallen, and Riedel (1981) conducted an assessment at least 10 years post retention of Sixty-five cases previously treated in the permanent-dentition stage with traditional edgewise mechanics, and retention

The sample was limited to first-premolar-extraction cases which had undergone routine edgewise orthodontic therapy followed by retention and eventual removal of all retention devices. Sixty-five cases with complete records before treatment, at the end of treatment, and a minimum of 10 years out of retention were collected.

The following conclusions were reached

1. Long-term alignment was variable and unpredictable.

2. No descriptive characteristics, such as Angle class, length of retention, age at the initiation of treatment, or sex, and no measured variables, such as initial or end-of-active-treatment alignment, overbite, overjet, arch width, or arch length, were of value in predicting the long-term result.

3. Arch dimensions i.e. width and length typically decreased after retention whereas crowding increased. This occurred in spite of treatment maintenance of initial intercanine width, treatment expansion, or constriction.

4. Success at maintaining satisfactory mandibular anterior alignment is less than 30 percent, with nearly 20 percent of the cases likely to show marked crowding many years after removal of retainers.

10

Årtun, Krogstad, Little (1990) conducted a study to determine if mandibular incisors could be proclined markedly without increasing the potential for relapse of crowding.

Sixty two Patients with surgically treated mandibular prognathism were selected. In twenty nine patients the mandibular incisors were proclined more than 10 degrees during the pre surgical orthodontic phase. The remaining thirty three patients had only minimal change in incisor inclination. A long-term follow-up examination was performed. Study casts were measured before and after treatment and three years after surgery. Cephalograms were evaluated before and after treatment, immediately before and after surgery, and three years after surgery.

Prior to therapy the patients treated with pre-surgical proclination had less dental arch length with more retroclined and crowded mandibular incisors than the patients in the other group. Dental arch length and intercanine width decreased and incisor irregularity increased in both groups during the follow-up periods. No inter group differences in changes were observed.

Lopez-Gavito et al (1985) evaluated the long-term response of the anterior open-bite malocclusion in forty-one white subjects who had undergone orthodontic treatment and were out of retention a minimum of 9 years 6 months. The purpose of the study was threefold: Changes occurring across time in the open-bite patients were analyzed by computer means using pre-treatment, post treatment, and long-term cephalometric radiographs and dental casts. More than 35% of the treated open-bite patients demonstrated a postretention open bite of 3 mm or more, with the relapse subgroup demonstrating across-time, less mandibular anterior dental height, less upper anterior facial height, greater lower anterior facial height, and less posterior facial height. Neither the magnitude of pre-treatment open bite, mandibular plane angle, nor any other single parameter of dentofacial form proved to be a reliable predictor of post treatment stability.

Little, Riedel, and Årtun (1988) Assessed pre-treatment, end of treatment, 10-year postretention, and 20-year postretention records of 31 four premolar extraction cases to evaluate stability and relapse of mandibular anterior alignment. The sample was limited to cases that had undergone edgewise orthodontic treatment followed by retention and eventual removal of retainers.

The summed displacement of the six lower anterior teeth, the Irregularity Index as described by Little, was determined for each mandibular cast. Crowding continued to increase during the 10- to 20-year postretention phase but to a lesser degree than from the end of retention to 10 years postretention. Only 10% of the cases were judged to have clinically acceptable mandibular alignment at the last stage of diagnostic records.

McReynolds and Little (1991) did a descriptive and comparative study of the stability of Intervention during the mixed dentition by serial extraction of deciduous teeth along with enucleation of second premolars or later second premolar extraction after full eruption in the permanent dentition. The dental casts and cephalometric radiographs of 46 patients, treated with mandibular second premolar extraction and edgewise orthodontic mechanotherapy, were evaluated for changes over a minimum 10-year postretention period. Arch length and arch width decreased with time and incisor irregularity increased

12

throughout the postretention period. No predictors or associations could be found to help the clinician in determining the long-term prognosis in terms of stability.

Little and Riedel (1989) Evaluated the alignment of mandibular arches a minimum of 10 years after complete cessation of retainer wear in cases with pre-treatment spacing in the anterior part of the arch and a lack of crowding in the canine and premolar area. The clinical hypothesis to be tested was that such cases usually show closure of spacing along with minimal future crowding and would therefore require minimal retention or no retention.

Consistent reduction of arch length and intercanine width into adult years was seen. Intercanine width constriction typically occurred while arch length decreased in every case, both width and length reduction being progressive with time. Crowding was minimal for the majority of cases; few demonstrated the severe crowding more typical of cases with pre-treatment crowding.

Riedel, Little and Bui (1992) evaluated the stability of cases treated by extracting one or two mandibular incisors. Pre-treatment, post treatment and 10-year postretention dental cast and lateral cephalogram records of 42 patients were evaluated. Each patient had undergone edgewise orthodontic treatment following removal of one or two mandibular incisors and various maxillary teeth. This result was considerably more favorable than the results of previously reported premolar extraction cases. Intercanine width decreased during treatment and continued to decrease postretention in most cases. Overbite and overjet remained acceptable. No associations could be found to predict the amount of relapse.

Elms, Buschang, Alexander (1996) evaluated the face-bow therapy, in conjunction with full-fixed appliance therapy, of 42 patients. Treatment goals had been attained for all patients. The results showed that mandibular and maxillary arch widths were increased significantly during treatment. Mandibular intercanine width decreased 0.3 mm during the postretention period; the remaining width measures increased or remained stable. Arch length, which did not change during treatment, decreased 1.0mm after treatment. Overjet and overbite decreased 4.4mm and 2.5mm, respectively, during treatment. Both overjet (0.5mm) and overbite (0.4mm) showed small increases after retention. Mandibular incisor irregularity was decreased 2.7 mm during treatment and increased only 0.4mm after treatment. Within the limits of the study, it was concluded that, when the described techniques are used, non-extraction therapy for patients with Class II malocclusion is largely stable.

Sadowsky and Sakols (1982) evaluated the long-term stability of orthodontic treatment in a group of ninety-six former patients who were treated between 12 and 35 years previously. Ninety of the ninety-six cases were within the ideal range at the end of treatment. Most of the cases showed an improvement of their malocclusions in the long-term stage. However, of the ninety-six subjects, sixty-nine (72 %) had at least one variable outside the ideal range in the long-term follow-up. A moderately increased overjet and

14

overbite was responsible in most instances for the result being outside the ideal range in the long term. The long-term result as compared to the original malocclusion exhibited increased overbite in 16 percent of the cases, increased mandibular anterior crowding in 9 percent of the cases, and increased overjet in 5 percent of the cases.

Suggested contributing factors

Third molars

Early and current literature cites the third molar as a contributory factor to relapse after orthodontic treatment has been completed. It is also thought to contribute to the occurrence or aggravation of crowding of late lower anterior crowding. According to Schwarze prophylactic germectomy of the third molar after orthodontic treatment should lessen subsequent crowding of the lower incisors.

 There have thus been a number of studies aimed at ascertaining whether the third molars contribute to the occurrence or aggravation of crowding, but the significance of the presence of the third molar has not as yet been clearly established. The fact that the results are controversial may, as several authors have pointed out, be due to the third molar being only one among a number of causative factors.

Lindqvist and Thilander (1982) conducted a study to ascertain whether the lower third molar, in combination with other variables such as facial morphology and space conditions, can contribute to the occurrence or aggravation of crowding. The subjects consisted of twenty-three boys and twenty-nine girls with impacted third molars on both sides of the mandible. The impacted molar on one side was removed, while the other, nonextracted side was used as a control. Average age at the time of operation was 15.5 years (range, 13 to 19). Close to the operation and annually for at least 3 years afterward, study casts and cephalograms (lateral, frontal, and oblique) were taken. The findings indicated that (1) despite analyses of many variables, this study has not been able to predict

16

which patients should react favorably or unfavorably to removal of the third lower molars in cases of anticipated crowding; (2) in cases with severe crowding removal of the molars could be recommended; (3) correct proximal contacts seem to be of importance in keeping the space that is achieved by extraction, while incorrect ones may spoil it

Shanley (1962) conducted a study to determine what influence mandibular third molars have on mandibular anterior teeth.

Forty – four subjects were divided into three groups – bilaterally impacted, erupted and congenitally absent mandibular third molars. No patients exhibited edentulous areas anterior to the third molars in the mandible.

The crowding of the six mandibular anterior teeth was determined by measuring, on plaster casts, the available arch circumference for these six teeth and subtracting the sum of the mesiodistal diameters of the six teeth. A positive value indicated spacing and a negative value indicated crowding. The procumbency of the mandibular incisors was measured from lateral cephalometric roentgenograms.

There was no significant difference between the means of the crowding measurements in the three groups and no significant difference in the means of the angulation measurements in the three groups at the one percent level. This result would indicate that mandibular third molars exert little influence on crowding or procumbency of mandibular anterior teeth.

Kahl – Nieke, Fischbach, Schwarze (1995) analyzed post-retention changes and to reveal factors which may pay a role as predictors for long-term prognosis. Pre-treatment, end-of-treatment, and post-retention models of 226 cases with all types of anomaly were used to measure intercanine and intermolar width, arch length, and sum of the mesiodistal dimension of the incisors, irregularity index, crowding, molar and canine relationship, overjet, and overbite.

1.   Many years after orthodontic treatment, a large number of cases exhibited an increase in lower crowding which was outside the ideal range. Relapse of maxillary crowding and mandibular anterior irregularity occurred in nearly half the sample.

2.   Pre-treatment variables such as increased mesiodistal incisor dimension, severe crowding and incisor irregularity, arch length deficiency, intermolar and intercanine constriction, and increased overbite were found to be associated factors in the process of post-retention increase of crowding and incisor irregularity.

3.   The amount of therapeutic increase in upper and lower intermolar width was found to be a factor in mandibular incisor relapse, which occurred more often in cases with 'over treated' arch width.

4.   The extraction subgroup exhibited significantly more relapse of crowding and rotations than the non-extraction sample.

5.   Post-treatment spacing, arch expansion, increased arch length, and residual Class II or III molar relationships were found to be associated with changes in incisor alignment.

6.   Lower arch crowding was found to be influenced by the presence of third molars to a minor degree: when lower third molars were missing, mandibular teeth showed (statistically) significantly less relapse of crowding than those cases with impacted or erupted third molars. However, the clinical relevance of this finding remains questionable.

Kaplan (1974) conducted a study to investigate whether the mandibular third molars have a significant influence on post – treatment changes in the mandibular dental arch and on anterior crowding relapse. A sample of seventy five orthodontically treated Caucasian patients an average of 9.3 years out of retention with a mean post – eruption age of 26.6 years was collected, thirty patients had bilaterally erupted mandibular third molars and 25 had bilateral third molar agenesis.

Dental casts (Pre-treatment, End-of active treatment and post retention dental casts were examined to assess the change in mandibular arch dimensions and crowding and rotation of lower anterior teeth. Cephalometric investigations evaluated changes in lower incisor and lower first molar positions. The following conclusions were reached.

During the post-treatment period no significant differences were apparent in the changes in arch length, lower incisor position, or lower incisor axial inclination between the different groups. It did not appear that third molars had any significant influence upon post treatment changes in arch length, lower molar position, lower incisor position or lower axial inclination or on dimensional changes in intercanine and intermolar widths.

Margaret Richardson (1996) compared Skeletal and dental morphology, and related growth changes during a 3 – year period following second permanent molar eruption, in a group of 21 subjects who had no increase in lower arch crowding, with another group of 21 subjects whose lower arch crowding had increased by 1.0 mm or more during the same period.

This investigation suggests that a mesially directed force is the most important cause of increased lower arch crowding in the early teenage years.

1. Mesial migration of molars and an increase in the inter-incisal angle are associated with an increase in lower arch crowding between the ages of 12.5 and 15.5 years.

2. The investigation did not support the view that a particular type of skeletal morphology or a specific pattern of growth is associated with an increase in lower arch crowding at this time.

Ades et al (1990) conducted a study to determine the relationship of third molars to changes in the mandibular dental arch. The sample for this study consisted of four groups and subgroups. The groups consisted of premolar extraction treated, nonextraction treated with initial generalized spacing, nonextraction treated, and serial extraction untreated subjects. The subgroups were divided into persons who had mandibular third molars that were either impacted, erupted into function, congenitally absent, or extracted at least 10 years before postretention records.

The mean postretention time interval was 13 years, with a range of 10 to 28 years. The mean postretention age was 28 years 6 months, with a range of 18 years 6 months to 39 years 4 months. Two-way analysis of variance with repeated measures was used to compare the changes over time (before treatment, at end of active treatment, and after retention) of groups and third molar subgroups. With time, mandibular incisor irregularity increased while arch length and intercanine width decreased. The eruption patterns of mandibular incisors and first molars were similarly dispersed in all groups studied. The findings between the subgroups in which mandibular third molars were impacted, erupted into function, congenitally absent, or extracted 10 years before postretention records revealed no significant differences between any of the subgroups for the parameters studied.

No significant differences in mandibular growth were found between the third molar subgroups; this suggests that **persons with third molars erupted into satisfactory function do not have a significantly different mandibular growth pattern than those whose third molars are impacted or congenitally missing.** In the majority of cases some degree of mandibular incisor crowding took place after retention, but this change was not significantly different between third molar subgroups. This finding suggests that **the recommendation for mandibular third molar removal with the objective of alleviating or preventing mandibular incisor irregularity may not be justified.**

Continuing growth

Nanda and Nanda (1992) in their article Dentofacial growth in long-term retention and stability noted that many patients at the completion of orthodontic treatment may still be going through the pubertal growth spurt, and there may be others who have not even entered the period of accelerated pubertal growth. This observation is of particularly greater significance in boys than in girls, since boys generally mature later.

They stated that hence, failure to recognize the continuing effect of dentofacial growth after the completion of orthodontic treatment and its resultant favourable or unfavourable effects on the physiognomy and its dental relationships may jeopardize long-term stability of the orthodontic result. They said the convenient assumption is often made by the clinician at the completion of treatment that future skeletal growth is of no consequence or that dentofacial changes will be proportional and thus will maintain the skeletal relationships that were established during treatment. Therefore the major focus during retention is placed on maintenance of the corrected positions of the teeth, and no compensations are made for the future dentoalveolar and skeletal growth of the jaws in either the horizontal or the vertical direction.

They suggested that the retention devices should be differentially selected on the basis of dentofacial morphology and the anticipated magnitude and directions of growth instead of simply using the clinician's favourite procrustean-bed retention appliance for all cases and that the answer to the question of long-term stability is long-term retention— dynamic, not static.

Change in arch form, intercanine width

De La Cruz et al (1995) conducted a study to evaluate the long-term stability of orthodontically induced changes in maxillary and mandibular arch form. Dental casts were evaluated before treatment, after treatment, and a minimum of 10 years after retention for 45 patients with Class I and 42 Class II, Division 1 malocclusions who received four first premolar extraction treatment. Computer generated arch forms were used to assess changes in arch shape over time. Findings demonstrated a rounding of arch form during treatment followed by a change to a more tapered form. Arch form tended to return toward the pre-treatment shape after retention. The greater the treatment change, the greater the tendency for postretention change. However, individual variation was considerable. The patient's pre-treatment arch form appeared to be the best guide to future arch form stability, but minimizing treatment change was no guarantee of postretention stability.

Shapiro (1974) conducted an evaluation of the stability of the mandibular dental arch in orthodontically treated cases 10 years after retentive appliances were removed. Changes in mandibular intercanine width, intermolar width and arch length were examined and it was determined whether a significant relationship existed between these variables and Angles classification and extraction therapy.

He found that mandibular intercanine demonstrated a strong tendency to return to its pre treatment dimension in all groups. Mandibular arch length decreased substantially in every group during the post retention period.

In non-extraction cases intermolar width was maintained throughout treatment and decreased post treatment. In the extraction cases intermolar width decreased during treatment and continued to decrease post treatment.

Moussa, O'Reilly, and Close (1995) evaluated the long-term changes of maxillary and mandibular dental arch measurements in patients who were treated with the soft tissue-borne palatal expander and edgewise appliances. Changes in intercanine width, intermolar width, arch length, arch perimeter, and Irregularity Index were examined. The sample comprised of 165 dental casts randomly selected from patients who had been out of retention for 8 to 10 years at a mean age of 30 years. Measurements were made directly on dental casts obtained at the three time intervals: before treatment, after treatment, and after retention. Treatment with the rapid palatal expander presented good stability for upper intercanine width, upper and lower intermolar widths and incisor irregularity. Lower intercanine, arch length and perimeter presented poor stability.

Bishara et al (1973) investigated the stability of maxillary and mandibular intercanine width and the relapse experienced in overbite and overjet. Thirty orthodontically treated cases all requiring 1st premolar extraction and edgewise mechanics, were assessed before treatment, following treatment and after a minimum retention period of 6 months. Measurements used were overbite, overjet, intercanine width and mandibular plane angle. They concluded that relapse is a reality in intercanine width and in overjet – overbite correction.

Tooth dimensions and position

Peck and Peck (1972) presented data which indicated that the presence or absence of lower incisor crowding was related to the shape of the lower anterior teeth. Persons with ideal incisor alignment were shown to have incisors with smaller mesiodistal and larger labiolingual (faciolingual) dimensions than persons with incisor crowding. On the basis of these findings, they suggested clinical guidelines. They determined the maximum desirable values for the ratio Mesiodistal width / Labiolingual width multiplied by 100 to be 88 to 92 for a central incisor and 90 to 95 for a lateral incisor. When the ratio exceeded these values, reproximation ("stripping") was indicated to reduce the mesiodistal dimension, thereby altering the ratio so that it was in the favorable range for long-term postretention stability of the lower anterior segment.

Smith, Davidson, and Gipe (1982) addressed the question of whether or not lower incisor tooth shapes, i.e. the mesiodistal width divided by labiolingual width, which have been proposed as important factors in lower incisor crowding, are more useful than simple measurements of incisor mesiodistal length.

They found that the use of tooth size measurements or ratios as a guide to clinical procedures is an oversimplification of a complex problem.

Keane and Engle (1979) in a study to find correlations between mesiodistal incisor size and specific craniofacial measurements taken from lateral and frontal head films found the post treatment stability of the lower incisor to be a function of the relationship of lower incisor size to the size of the face and jaws. Cases which could accommodate wider incisors possess greater values for corpus length and mandibular arc and lower mandibular plane angles demonstrating brachycephalic characteristics. Those patients who cannot accommodate wide incisors show smaller measurements for the above variables and a dolicocephalic pattern.

Gilmore and Little (1984) Examined 164 cases from the records of the University Of Washington Department Of Orthodontics, out of which 134 had been orthodontically treated and with a minimum of 10 years of retention. Measurements were made from the postretention plaster casts and from serial cephalometric head films.

Statistical tests showed that there was a weak association between incisor widths and irregular alignment over the long term. Mean dimensional differences between crowded and uncrowded incisors were small in the few pooled or segregated groups in which statistically significant differences were found. When incisor dimensions were combined with pretreatment, post-treatment, or long-term cephalometric and cast measurements, only weak and not clinically useful associations were found with long-term incisor alignment.

While there was a weak tendency for narrower incisors to be associated with better alignment, or a greater mesiodistal dimension to be associated with crowding, the association is so weak that reduction of the widths of incisors to fit a specific range cannot be expected to produce a stable alignment. Narrower mesiodistal widths of mandibular incisors did not ensure long-term stability in orthodontically treated cases.

Siatkowski (1974) assessed the role of lingual uprighting of the lower incisors as an etiologic factor in the lower anterior crowding seen in the post – orthodontic treatment period and found that during late growth changes in anterior arch width and depth result in a decrease in anterior arch circumference, greater on average in the mandibular than in the maxillary arch. The decrease in anterior arch depth can be fully accounted for by lingual uprighting of the incisors.

Relapse in the transverse dimension

Rapid palatal expansion (RPE) is the technique of choice to correct skeletal maxillary transverse deficiency. RPE is characterized by a widening of the midpalatal suture by forcing a lateral shift of the two horizontal processes of the maxilla. Such widening, however, is not uniformly equal, it is greater in the anterior than the posterior segment, forming a V-shaped expansion of the suture in the horizontal plane. It is well-documented that even after a retention period the expanded upper dental arch has a strong tendency to rebound to its previous form.

Zimring and Isaacson studied the nature of relapse associated with RPE they stated that retention of rapid maxillary expansion cases would not necessarily depend on the presence of bone in the opened midpalatal suture, but rather on the creation of a stable relationship at the articulations of the maxilla and the other bones of the facial skeleton. As long as forces remain at adjacent maxillary articulations, there is no reason to assume that bone deposited within the midpalatal void would not be resorbed in the reestablishment of a physiologic equilibrium.

The residual loads acting upon the appliance at the end of the expansion phase of treatment were shown to entirely dissipate within a five to seven week period As the expansion screw was stabilized with brass ligature wire, only two possibilities explained the decrease in load (release of potential energy) during fixed retention: 1) further displacement of the maxillary segments can occur or 2) the teeth involved in supporting the appliance move independently of the skeletal structures. Although it is probable that a combination of both factors occurs, it is apparent from studies using implants that skeletal repositioning predominates until late in retention when the loads have decreased to physiologic levels more conducive to orthodontic tooth movement. Whether the skeletal repositioning that occurs is traumatic or is due to a physiologic reorganization of the contiguous maxillary sutures is a question for further study. The lack of dimensional changes incident to appliance removal following the retention period was interpreted as evidence that a stable relationship between the maxilla and the other bones of the facial skeletal had been created. The slight variable decrease in inter bicuspid and intermolar dimension observed ten and thirty days after all retention had been discontinued may be attributed to the influences of the muscular drape, facets of occlusion and relapse of the portion of the expansion contributed by orthodontic tooth movement.

Furthermore, it appears that the length of time required for skeletal readjustment during retention is dependent upon the amount of residual load remaining at the termination of appliance activation, as the rate of load decay was essentially constant for all patients. Using a slower activation schedule, and thereby avoiding the accumulation of large residual loads, the retention phase of treatment may be significantly shortened while the total treatment time would remain essentially the same. Following this procedure may have its advantages in being less traumatic and thereby evoking a more physiologic response from the involved tissues.

The maximum relapse potential of the involved skeletal elements is evaluated according to the loads remaining on the expansion appliance at any particular moment. If these remaining loads prove to be active through specific measurable distances, which seems reasonable, judicious overexpansion to compensate for a predictable amount of relapse may also shorten the period of fixed retention and thereby allow conventional orthodontic therapy to be instituted at an earlier date.

Vardimon et al investigated the mineralization pattern of the midpalatal suture after rapid palatal expansion was attempted in 10 treated and 2 control cats, in light of the tendency of RPE to relapse. The rapid palatal expansion treatment consisted of active expansion (25 days), retention (60 days), and relapse (60 days) phases. Standardized occlusal radiographs were taken periodically and analyzed for suture width, suture optical density in anterior vs. posterior regions, and suture area measurements of radiopaque vs. radiolucent zones. Nine cats exhibited suture splitting. During the active phase, the radiolucent zone (nonmineralized tissue) increased 12-fold and the increase in optical density was 50% greater in the anterior over the posterior suture region, demonstrating increased formation of loose connective tissue at the anterior region. During the retention period, the suture's radio opaque zone (mineralized tissue) increased by 62%, the radiolucent zone declined (64%) and the suture width decreased (65%) indicating reorganization of mineralized tissue.

The decrease in optical density (increased mineralization) was 2.5 times greater in the posterior over the anterior suture region, indicating that the remineralization (closure) pattern of the expanded suture is analogous to a zipper closed in a posteroanterior direction.

They extrapolated that the retention of the suture anterior region should be longer than the posterior region to catch up the lag in rebuilding and maturation of the newly deposited hard tissue.

It was found that 78% of the animals clearly showed a relapse reaction, therefore extending the retention phase was found to be imperative for further rebuilding of hard tissue and for completion of the maturation of the newly deposited hard tissue. They concluded that to counteract the pressure of the facial musculature, a certain amount of calcified bone must be formed in the callus of bony fracture or bone grafting must be added into maxillary osteotomies, or calcified tissue must be laid at the margins of the expanded surface.

Vardimon et al studied the influence of RPE in cats with synostosed sutures, they examined sutural displacement (S_d-S_d), tooth tip (T_t-T_t), tooth displacement (T_d-T_d), and alveolar process tipping and bending $(A_{t+b}-A_{t+b})$. The involvement of these four components was studied on 10 rapid palatal expansion treated and two control cats during an active phase (25 days), a retention phase (60 days), and a relapse phase (60 days). The midpalatal suture was analyzed for linear measurements, radiopaque versus radiolucent zones and optical density from occlusal radiographs.

In patent suture (animals with sutural split), optical density increased during rapid palatal expansion (soft tissue build-up) and decreased during retention (remineralization) and relapse phases (medical convergence of the palatal processes). In the animal without sutural split, a continuous decrease in the optical density (predetermined ossification) was found.

- The strong involvement of tooth displacement as against sutural displacement in the synostosed suture highlighted the high probability of obtaining fenestration or dehiscence, or even complete perforation of the anchored roots through the buccal cortical plate if RPE treatment is applied in nonpatent midpalatal suture.

- Severe residual forces were apparently stored in the system in sutural synostosis, giving rise to continuous expansion of the intercanine distance during the entire retention phase.

- Sutural mineralization is generated during the retention phase.

- Extrapolating the results of the study suggests that the anterior sutural region required a two fold longer retention period than the posterior to complete sutural mineralization.

Retention

Retention is the phase of orthodontic treatment which maintains the teeth in their orthodontically corrected positions following the cessation of active orthodontic tooth movement. Orthodontic retainers resist the tendency of teeth to return to their pre-treatment positions under the influence of periodontal, occlusal and soft tissue forces, and continuing dentofacial growth. Very few prospective controlled studies have evaluated the effectiveness of retention. Retention is advisable for almost all treated malocclusions. Recent trends found that the most commonly used retention period was 12 months.[1] This approach is supported by histological studies which have shown that the supracrestal periodontal fibres remain stretched and displaced for more than 7 months after the cessation of orthodontic tooth movement,[2,3] suggesting that the retention period should generally be at least 7 months. However, individual patient factors can often modify the length of the retention phase.

Occlusal and other factors which may modify the retention protocol

Lower incisor alignment

Increases in lower incisor irregularity occur throughout life in a large proportion of patients following orthodontic treatment and also in untreated subjects. Recent evidence suggests that most change will take place by the middle of the third decade.[4] It has been suggested that prolonged retention of the lower labial segment until the end of facial growth may reduce the severity of lower incisor crowding.[5] Patients' expectations of the stability of their lower incisor alignment should be considered on completion of orthodontic treatment. If an individual is unwilling to accept any deterioration in lower incisor alignment following orthodontic treatment then permanent fixed or removable retention may have to be considered.

Deterioration in lower incisor alignment during the second, third and fourth decades of life has been reported in multiple studies of normal subjects, and subjects with previous orthodontic treatment followed by retention.[19,20] Such changes in lower labial segment alignment are now recognized to be a normal rather than exceptional occurrence and occur throughout life, although it is reported that the greatest changes in untreated occlusions occur before the age of 18 years.[4,21,22] The use of prolonged retention of the lower labial segment has been suggested to be effective in reducing the severity of lower incisor crowding following treatment. The results reported by Sadowsky et al[5] using an average period of 8.4 years with a fixed lower lingual retainer were more favourable than other studies using shorter retention times. However no comparative studies have been reported.

Corrected rotations of anterior teeth

As the supracrestal gingival fibres are known to take the longest amount of time to reorganize, prolonged retention of corrected rotations may be helpful in reducing relapse. While the use of adjunctive circumferential supracrestal fiberotomy has been shown to be effective in reducing relapse within the first 4-6 years after debonding, the additional long term clinical benefit from the procedure is relatively small.[6]

The pattern of rotational tooth displacements in a malocclusion has a strong tendency to repeat itself when post treatment changes occur.[23] Edwards[6] observed that most relapse in rotations occurred within 4-6 years of appliance removal.

Changes in the antero-posterior lower incisor position

Any intentional or non-intentional change of more than 2mm indicates the need for long-term or indefinite retention.[7] Opinions differ about the amount of stable proclination of the lower incisors that can be achieved during orthodontic treatment.[24,25] Mills[26] found that following orthodontic treatment the average amount of stable proclination of the lower incisors was 1-2 mm. Houston and Edler[27] reported that when the antero-posterior position of the lower incisors was changed during treatment, in the majority of cases the lower incisors returned towards their pre-treatment position after retention. Thus the consensus of evidence supports the view that excessive lower incisor proclination should be avoided unless prolonged retention is planned.

Correction of deep overbite

Following the correction of a very deep overbite, the use of an anterior bite-plane until the completion of facial growth has been recommended.[7] This may be particularly useful when there is evidence of an anterior mandibular growth rotation.[8]

Correction of anterior open bites

While the use of retainers incorporating posterior bite-blocks has been recommended for prolonged retention of anterior open bite malocclusions with unfavourable growth patterns[7], there is currently a lack of scientific evidence to support this. The stability of anterior open bite correction is unpredictable, with one study reporting that more than one third of cases relapsed to more than 3mm anterior open bite when examined a minimum of nine years following retention.[28] No predictors of relapse could be identified. Although bite-block retainers are commonly advocated for treated anterior open bite cases, no controlled studies of their effectiveness have been published.

Patients with a history of periodontal disease or root resorption

In patients with previously treated severe periodontal disease, permanent retention is advised. For those with minimum to moderate disease, a more routine retention protocol can be used.[9] There is evidence of an increased risk of deterioration of lower incisor alignment post-retention in cases with root resorption or crestal bone loss.[10] These cases may therefore benefit from prolonged retention.

Growth modification treatment

Following the use of headgear or functional appliances, retention using a modified activator appliance has been reported as effective in maintaining Class II correction.[11] However, no comparative studies have confirmed the usefulness of this form of retention.

Correction of posterior and anterior cross-bites

When the incisor overbite and posterior intercuspation are adequate for maintaining the correction, no retention is necessary.[12]

36

Adult Patients

When the periodontal supporting tissues are normal and no occlusal settling is required, there is no evidence to support any changes in retention protocol for adult patients compared with adolescent patients.

Spaced dentitions

Permanent retention has been recommended following orthodontic treatment to close generalized spacing or a midline diastema in an otherwise normal occlusion.[13] Post-retention treatment results in adults with similar retention protocols have been shown to be at least as stable as those in adolescents with regard to all clinically relevant factors including midline alignment, overjet, overbite, molar relationship and incisor alignment.[29,30] In addition, Richardson[4,21,22] has shown that most deterioration in lower incisor alignment occurs during late adolescence and early adulthood with the changes above the age of 21 being much less marked.

Kaplan (1988) following a review of views and studies on retention that the most defensible logical position to take in the overall retention program to be Initiated is that the decision for the duration of retention appliances (of all but a small number of cases) should be within the option of the informed patient or the patient's parent, as well as the orthodontist, for the following reasons. First, the patient and parent (if the patient is a minor) have or should have been informed of the previously summarized "bad" news of the relapse statistics as far as comprehension permits.

He then proceeds to give guidelines on retention procedures:

1. There are very few cases requiring minimum or no retaining appliances and these would include:

a. Blocked out canines in Class I extraction cases with no incisor crowding

b. Class I anterior and/or posterior crossbites with very steep cusps and no anterior crowding

c. Class II cases slightly overtreated with headgear to restrict maxillary growth with sufficient arch length indicated by mandibular anterior spacing and absolutely no mandibular incisor rotations

d. The above-described cases should be seen on a scheduled basis during the posttreatment adolescent period to check possible spacing or unfavorable growth changes or TMJ symptoms.

2. Routine cases, extraction or nonextraction, should have retaining appliances— fixed or removable.

a. At least until the destiny of the third molar teeth is determined [or]

b. Until the growth process has slowed in late teens and early twenties [and]

c. Afterward at the option of the patient

3. Cases that will need indefinite retention

a. Class II, Division 2 Angle deep bite cases

b. Arch expansion treatment for esthetic demands

c. Patients with uncontrolled muscular or tongue habits

d. Again the orthodontist should be most emphatic about this need.

4. Cases that require operative procedures with indefinite retention

a. Treatment limitations such as tooth size discrepancies (that is, larger maxillary teeth) may result in increased overbite or super Class I.

b. Reversely, larger mandibular teeth will result in end-to-end incisor relationships, maxillary spacing, or buccal end-on occlusion.

c. Stripping or reproximation of oversized teeth and esthetic bonding of malshaped or undersized teeth may help resolve this problem.

d. A very vertical incisal relationship, which for any reason cannot be corrected, will lead to deepening overbite unless retained.

e. The patient should be informed.

5. Cases requiring special construction and/or renewal of removable retaining appliances or acrylic on the labial bows

a. Posttreatment adolescent palatal changes

b. Late mandibular growth spurt and Tweed type C growers

c. To maintain torque and overbite correction

6. The orthodontist can never be completely certain that the individual case will be in the 33% that will not relapse, even if only mildly, if all or a majority of the aforementioned rules, factors, or so-called principles pertaining to stability have not been violated.

7. The patient should be apprised of the expected changes of the maturing dentition, especially of mandibular and maxillary crowding (the "smile winners" study in California and late mandibular incisor crowding in untreated normal occlusions.

His answer to the question of why and when the patient should be given the option of almost indefinite retention is as follows:

(1) when the orthodontist accepts the present limitation of definitive knowledge of the aforementioned multiplicity of the factors that pertain to stability in the individual cases and

(2) when the patient has been advised of the statistics (66%) of relapse in well-treated cases and elects or prefers long-range retention.

It is not a passive role for the patient or the orthodontist. To check appliance fit and health of the supporting tissues, the patient should be monitored on an agreed upon schedule. There is a decreasing frequency of appointments for the first 2 to 3 years and after than an annual visit should suffice. An occlusion that can change because of untoward dynamic forces should not only be guarded by retainer but, where indicated, by stripping, circumferential supracrestal fiberotomy, and orthognathic surgery. This retention procedure will maintain desirable anterior tooth alignment, overbite, proximal contact, overjet, axial inclination, arch form, cuspal relationship, and an optimum defense against possible TMJ problems for a considerable portion of the patient's life.

Removable retainers

Proffit (1998) in his book *Contemporary Orthodontics* states that Removable appliances can serve effectively for retention against intra-arch instability and are also useful as retainers (in the form of modified functional appliances or part-time headgear) in patients with growth problems.

Hawley Retainers

By far the most common removable retainers is the Hawley retainer, designed in the 1920s as an active removable appliance. It incorporates clasps on molar teeth and a characteristic outer bow with adjustment loops, spanning from canine to canine. Because it covers the palate, it automatically provides a potential bite plane to control overbite.

The ability of this retainer to provide some tooth movement was a particular asset with fully banded fixed appliances, since one function of the retainer was to close band spaces between the incisors, and it was sometimes modified to use elastics for this purpose. With bonded appliances on the anterior teeth or after using a tooth positioner for finishing, there is no longer any need to close spaces with a retainer. However, the outer bow provides excellent control of the incisors even if it is not adjusted to retract them.

When first premolars have been extracted, one function of a retainer is to keep the extraction space closed, which the standard design of the Hawley retainer cannot do. Even worse, the standard Hawley labial bow extends across a first premolar extraction space, tending to wedge it open. A common modification of the Hawley retainer for use in extraction cases is a bow soldered to the buccal section of Adams clasps on the first molars, so that the action of the bow helps hold the extraction site closed. Alternative designs for extraction cases are to wrap the labial bow around the entire arch, using circumferential clasps on second molars for retention ; or to bring the labial wire from the baseplate between the lateral incisor and canine and to bend or solder a wire extension distally to control the canines. The latter alternative does not provide an active force to keep an extraction space closed, but avoids having the wire cross through the extraction site, and gives positive control of canines that were labially positioned initially (which the loop of the traditional Hawley design may not provide).

The clasp locations for a Hawley retainer must be selected carefully, since clasp wires crossing the occlusal table can disrupt rather than retain the tooth relationships established during treatment. Circumferential clasps on the terminal molar or lingual extension clasps may be preferred over the more effective Adams clasp if the occlusion is tight.

The palatal coverage of a removable place like the maxillary Hawley retainer makes it possible to incorporate a bite plane lingual to the upper incisors, to control bite depth. For any patient who once had an excessive overbite, light contact of the lower incisors against the baseplate of the retainer is desired.

Removable Wraparound Retainers

A second major type of removable orthodontic retainer is the wraparound or clip-on retainer, which consists of a plastic bar (usually wire-reinforced) along the labial and lingual surfaces of the teeth. A full-arch wraparound retainer firmly holds each tooth in position. This is not necessarily an advantage, since one object of a retainer should be to allow each tooth to move individually, stimulating reorganization of the PDL. In addition, a wraparound retainer, through quite esthetic, is often less comfortable than a Hawley retainer and may not be effective in maintaining overbite correction. A full-arch wraparound retainer is indicated primarily when periodontal breakdown requires splinting the teeth together.

Canine-to-canine clip-on retainer

A variant of the wraparound retainer is widely used in the lower anterior region. This appliance has the great advantage that it can be used to realign irregular incisors, if mild crowding has developed after treatment, but it is well tolerated as a retainer alone. An upper canine-to-canine wraparound occasionally is useful in adults with long clinical crowns but rarely is indicated and usually would not be tolerated in younger patients because of occlusal interferences.

In a lower extraction case, usually it is a good idea to extend a canine-to-canine wraparound distally on the lingual only to the central groove of the first molar. This provides control of the second premolar and the extraction site, but the retainer must be made carefully to avoid lingual undercuts in the premolar and molar region. Posterior extension of the lower retainer, of course, also is indicated when the posterior teeth were irregular before treatment.

Positioners

A tooth positioner also can be used as a removable retainer, either fabricated for this purpose alone, or more commonly, continued as a retainer after serving initially as a finishing device. Positioners are excellent finishing devices and under special circumstances can be used to an advantage as retainers. For routine use, however, a positioner does not make a good retainer. The major problems are:

1. The pattern of wear of a positioner does not match the pattern usually desired for retainers. Because of its bulk, patients often have difficulty wearing a positioner full-time or nearly so. In fact, positioners tend to be worn less than the

recommended 4 hours per day after the first few weeks, although they are reasonably well tolerated by most patients during sleep.

2. Positioners do not retain incisor irregularities and rotations as well as standard retainers. This problem follows directly from the first one : a retainer is needed nearly full-time initially to control intra-arch alignment. Also, overbite tends to increase while a positioner is being worn, and this effect as well probably relates in large part to the fact that it is worn only a small percentage of the time.

A positioner does have one major advantage over a standard removable or wraparound retainer, however – it maintains the occlusal relationships as well as intra-arch tooth positions. For a patient with a tendency toward Class III relapse, a positioner made with a tendency toward Class III relapse, a positioner made with the jaws rotated somewhat downward and backward may be useful. Although a positioner with the teeth set in a slightly exaggerated "supernormal" from the original malocclusion can be used for patients with a skeletal Class II or open bite growth pattern, it is less effective in controlling growth than part-time headgear or a functional appliance.

In fabricating a positioner, it is necessary to separate the teeth by 2 to 4mm. This means that an articulator mounting that records the patient's hinge axis is desirable. As a general guideline, the more the patient deviates from the average normal, and the longer the positioner will be worn, the more important it is to obtain an individualized hinge axis mounting on an adjustable articulator for positioner construction. If a positioner is to be used for only 2 to 4 weeks as a finishing device in a patient who will have some vertical growth during later retention, and if the patient has an approximately normal hinge axis, an individualized articulator mounting may be unnecessary. If a positioner is to be worn for many months as a retainer or if no growth can be anticipated, a precisely correct hinge axis becomes more important.

ACTIVE RETAINERS

"Active retainer" is a contradiction in terms, since a device cannot be actively moving teeth and serving as a retainer at the same time. It does happen, however, that relapse or growth changes after orthodontic treatment will lead to a need for some tooth movement during retention. This usually is accomplished with a removable appliance that continues as a retainer after it has repositioned the teeth, hence the name. A typical Hawley retainer, if used initially to close a small amount of band space, can be considered an active retainer, but the term usually is reserved for two specific situations: realignment of irregular incisors, and functional appliances to manage Class II or Class III relapse tendencies.

Realignment of Irregular Incisors: Spring Retainers

Recrowding of lower incisors is the major indication for an active retainer to correct incisor position. If late crowing has developed, it often is necessary to reduce the interproximal width of lower incisors before realigning them, so that the crowns do not tip labially into an obviously unstable position. The cause of the problem in these cases usually is late mandibular growth, which has uprighted the incisors, and they must be realigned in their more upright position. Not only does stripping of contacts reduce the Mesiodistal width of the incisors, decreasing the amount of space required for their alignment, it also flattens the contact areas, increasing the inherent stability of the arch in

45

this region. As with any procedure involving the modification of teeth, however, stripping must be done cautiously and judiciously. It is not indicated as a routine procedure.

Interproximal enamel can be removed with either abrasive strips or thin discs in a handpiece. Obviously, enamel reduction should not be overdone, but if necessary, the width of each lower incisor can be reduced upto 0.5mm on each side without going through the interproximal enamel. If an additional 2 mm of space can be gained, reducing each incisor 0.25mm per side, it is usually possible to realign typically crowded incisors.

If the irregularity is modest and if the teeth are to be realigned without moving facially, a canine-to-canine clip on is usually the active retainer used to realign crowded incisors. The steps in making such an active retainer are;

(1) reduce the interproximal width of the incisors and apply topical fluoride to the newly exposed enamel surfaces;

(2) prepare a laboratory model, on which the teeth can be reset into alignment; and

(3) fabricate a canine-to-canine clip-on appliance.

If there is more than a modest degree of relapse, however, placing a fixed appliance for comprehensive retreatment must be considered. With bonded brackets on the lower arch from premolar to premolar, superelastic NiTi wires can be used to bring the incisors back into alignment quite efficiently. If the incisors are advanced toward the lip when this is done, a bonded lingual retainer should be placed before the brackets are removed. Permanent retention obviously will be required after the realignment.

Essix thermoplastic copolyester retainers are a thinner, but stronger, cuspid-to-cuspid version of the full-arch, vacuum-formed devices. Advantages include:

46

- The ability to supervise without office visits.

- Absolute stability of the anterior teeth.

- Durability and ease of cleaning.

- Low cost and ease of fabrication.

- Minimal bulk and thickness (.015").

- The brilliant appearance of the teeth caused by light reflection.

A pressure-type thermoforming unit such as a Biostar is used to fabricate the appliance. Thermoplastic copolyester is used for the fabrication of Essix retainers. Thinner, . Copolyester, unlike polycarbonates, does not require heat treatment before thermoforming. It is much stronger, clearer, and resistant to abrasion than acrylic sheet, and thus produces thinner yet sturdier appliances.

Patient cast is positioned in the thermoforming unit so that the plastic will extend well into the facial and lingual gingivae. The casts are small enough that two or three retainers can be made from one sheet of Essix plastic. During the thermoforming, the thickness of the plastic is reduced from .030" to .015".

Surgical methods of retention

Edwards (1970) upon completion of rotational movement and 8 weeks of mechanical retention subjected all experimental teeth to a periodontal surgical procedure (circumferential supracrestal fiberotomy) in an attempt to alleviate the relapse tendency of the rotated teeth. This surgical technique consisted of inserting the point of a No. 11 Bard-Parker blade into the depth of the gingival sulcus and severing all fibrous attachments surrounding the tooth to a depth approximately 3 mm. below the crest of the alveolar bone.

Edwards (1988) also evaluated the efficacy of the circumferential supracrestal fiberotomy (CSF) procedure in alleviating dental relapse following orthodontic treatment. The surgical procedure appeared to be somewhat more effective in alleviating pure rotational relapse than in labiolingual relapse. On a long-term basis, the CSF procedure was shown to be more successful in reducing relapse in the maxillary anterior segment than in the mandibular anterior segment. Nevertheless, a significant and unpredictable variation in individual tooth movement following orthodontic treatment was observed in both the control and CSF groups.

Fricke, Christopher, Rankine (1996) studied the relapse tendency of orthodontically rotated teeth after electrosurgical circumferential fiberotomies and after conventional scalpel blade surgical procedures. Electrosurgical circumferential fiberotomies were performed on the designated second incisors, and circumferential fiberotomies with a scalpel blade were performed on the contralateral incisors. The teeth were retained for 1 month and relapse was measured 2 months pre retention.

The results of this study indicated that there was no significant difference in orthodontic relapse, gingival recession, and sulcus depth between the teeth treated with scalpel fiberotomies and those treated with electrosurgical fiberotomies. The data from this study demonstrate that electrosurgery was as effective as the conventional scalpel blade procedures in circumferential fiberotomies in dogs

Boese (1969) found that gingivectomy of orthodontically rotated teeth in dogs reduced the amount of subsequent relapse to one fourth that seen in rotated control teeth.

Stability of the rotated teeth was increased six fold by gingivectomy combined with an 8-week retention period. The pertinent facts were that gingivectomy of the rotated tooth, performed at the beginning of retention, reduced the amount of relapse which would occur otherwise, and the amount of reduction in relapse became significant when the rotated teeth were retained for at least 8 or 9 weeks. The effectiveness of gingivectomy was due to surgical removal of transseptal fibers which, even at the end of retention, remained stretched between the rotated and adjacent teeth.

If the gingivectomy is performed after only 4 weeks of retention, the principal fibers do not have sufficient time to complete their adjustment. Gingivectomy followed by a minimum of 8 weeks of retention significantly reduced relapse to one tenth its normal amount. A retention period of only 4 weeks masks the effectiveness of gingivectomy, because the first phase of relapse is still in progress.

49

Boese (1980) evaluated the long-term clinical results of CSF and reproximation on crowded mandibular arches which were orthodontically treated but never retained, and observed from 4 to 9 years post-treatment.

Observation of mandibular arches which had never been retained and observed 4-9 years after treatment provided dramatic evidence of stability in the mandibular anterior segment. This was reflected in the mean Irregularity Index of 9.18, S.D. 2.87 before treatment compared with a mean Irregularity Index of .62, S.D .37 post-treatment. Severe rotations which were present originally had not relapsed during the post-treatment period in contrast to other rotation studies where CSF was not used. Even those cases having marked bodily tooth displacement demonstrated exceptional stability which was confirmed by low post-treatment irregularity index scores

Based on the clinical findings of this study, the following conclusions were made:

1. Circumferential supracrestal fiberotomy (CSF) produced long-term stability of previously rotated teeth which were corrected orthodontically.

2. A slight overcorrection of tooth rotations should be accomplished at least six months prior to CSF to insure normal contact point relationships and principal fiber realignment.

3. Reproximation, precisely and conservatively performed, increased the long-term stability of the mandibular anterior segment.

4. The majority of all reproximation is performed early in treatment and within six months of band removal if no lower retention is employed.

5. Serial reproximation during the post-treatment period is often necessary, especially on patients experiencing marked horizontal growth or where lower arch

form has been significantly altered especially in the mandibular incisor-canine areas.

6.   The periodontium of those teeth which underwent CSF and reproximation displayed no significant increase in pocket depth, gingival recession, or loss of alveolar crestal bone, 4-9 years after treatment.

7.   The practice of not utilizing mandibular retention played an integral part in stabilizing the lower anterior segment.

Fixed retention

Fixed retention

Most recently the use of bonded fixed retainers has been introduced. Bonded fixed retainers consist of a length of orthodontic wire bonded to the teeth with acid-etch retained composite. At present three generations of fixed retainers are available.[1,3] These are:

- First generation-Plain blue Elgiloy wire with a loop at each terminal end for added retention

- Second generation- Similar diameter but multistranded wire

- Third generation—Round 0.032 inch stainless steel or 0.030 inch gold coated wire

Development of Bonded Retainers[1-7]

Kneirim published the first report of the use of this technique to construct bonded fixed retainers.

Early bonded fixed retainers were made with plain round or rectangular orthodontic wires, but Zachrisson[13] proposed the potential advantages for the use of multistranded wire and their construction. Artun and Zachrisson first described the clinical technique for the use of a multistranded wire canine-to-canine bonded fixed retainer. In this retainer the wire was bonded to the canine teeth only. In 1983, Zachrisson reported the use of multistranded wire in a bonded fixed retainer in which the wire was bonded to all the teeth in the labial segment. The proposed advantages of the use of multistranded wire are that the irregular surface offers increased mechanical retention for the composite without the need for the placement of retentive loops, and that the flexibility of the wire allows physiologic movement of the teeth, even when several adjacent teeth are bonded. As an alternative to multistranded wire, the use of resin fiberglass strips has been developed. The fiberglass strips are soaked in composite and bonded to acid-etched enamel. Although this technique has the advantage of reducing the bulk of the retainer, it has the disadvantage of creating a rigid splint, which limits physiologic tooth movement and contributes to a higher failure rate.

Indications for Bonded Retainers[34-37]

Lee considered the following to be indications for placement of a bonded canine-to-canine retainer:

- Severe pretreatment lower incisor crowding or rotation
- Planned alteration in the lower intercanine width
- After advancement of the lower incisors during active treatment
- After nonextraction treatment in mildly crowded cases
- After correction of deep overbite.

Zachrisson listed the following indications for clinical use of flexible wire retainer:

- Closed median diastema
- Spaced anterior teeth
- Adult cases with potential post orthodontic tooth migration
- Accidental loss of maxillary incisors, requiring closure, and retention of large anterior spaces
- Spacing reopening, after mandibular incisor extractions
- Severely rotated maxillary incisors
- Palatally impacted canines.

Techniques for Construction of Bonded Retainers[1-4]

Construction of bonded fixed retainer might appear to be simple, but if good long-term success is to be ensured, meticulous attention to detail is required. Two techniques have been described:

- Direct technique
- Indirect technique

Direct Technique:

The direct technique requires a length of wire to be prefabricated to accurately fit a recent cast. Loops are not required at the ends of the wire. The adaptation of the wire is checked clinically to ensure it locates passively against all tooth surfaces to be retained. The teeth are subsequently pumiced and acid etched as for direct bonding of orthodontic attachments. The wire is then accurately located on the teeth. At this point authors differ in their approach, and many methods for locating the wire have been described. These include the use of dental floss, orthodontic elastics, wire ligatures, wires tack welded to the retainer wire localizing devices, or fingers. It is recommended that a small amount of composite be used to tack the retainer in place at each end before adding the bulk of material. The composite can be shaped with an instrument dipped in unfilled resin or alcohol to produce the desired contour.

Indirect Technique:

The use of an indirect technique has been described to simplify the clinical procedure. The wire is prepared on the model, and inlay wax placed in the sites for the composite. A silicone impression material is placed over this and allowed to set. The wax is removed with boiling water. The teeth are prepared in the usual way and the composite is placed in the voids left by the wax. The impression complete with the retainer wire and composite is then placed over the teeth and held firmly in position until the composite has set. This indirect technique can be modified by placing composite directly on the model in place of the wax allowing the composite to set, then covering this with a vacuum-formed plastic sheet for subsequent location of the retainer in the mouth. In this technique, it is an unfilled resin-bonding agent that is then used to bond the retainer to the enamel.

Why fixed retention in some cases???[5-13]

The major cause of lower incisor crowding in the late teen years, is late growth of the mandible in the normal growth pattern. Especially if the lower incisors have previously been irregular, even a small amount of differential mandibular growth between ages 16 to 20 can cause crowding of these teeth. Relapse into crowding is almost always accompanied by lingual tipping of the central and lateral incisors in response to the pattern of growth. An excellent retainer to hold these teeth in alignment is a fixed lingual bar, attached only to the canines (or to canines and first premolars) and resting against the flat lingual surface of the lower incisors above the cingulum. This prevents the incisors from moving lingually and is also reasonably effective in maintaining correction of rotations in the incisor segment. Fixed canine to canine retainers must be made from a wire heavy enough to resist distortion over the rather long space between these teeth. Usually 30 mil steel is used for this purpose, with the end of the wire sandblasted to improve retention when it is bonded to the canines.

A second indication for a fixed retainer is situation where teeth must be permanently or semi-permanently bonded together to maintain the closure of a space between them. This is encountered most commonly when diastema between maxillary central incisor has been closed. Even if a frencectomy has been carried out, there is a tendency for a small space to open up between the upper central incisors. Since this is unsightly, prolonged or permanent retention usually is needed. The best retainer for this purpose is bonded section of flexible wire. The wire should be contoured so that it lies near the cingulum to keep it out of occlusal contact. The object of the retainer is to hold the teeth together while allowing them some ability to move independently during function, hence the importance of a flexible wire.

A fixed retainer is also the best choice to maintain a space where bridge, pontic or implant eventually will be place. Using a fixed retainer for a few months reduces mobility of the teeth and often makes it easier to place the fixed bridge that will serve, among other functions, as permanent orthodontic retainer. If further periodontal therapy is needed after the teeth have been positioned, several months or even years can pass before a bridge is placed, and a fixed retainer is definitely required. Implants should be place as soon as possible after the orthodontics is completed, so that integration of the implant can occur simultaneously with the initial stages of retention. It may be better in adults to bond a fixed retainer on the facial surface of posterior teeth when spaces have been closed.

The major objection to any fixed retainer is that it makes inter-proximal hygiene procedures more difficult. It is possible to floss between teeth that have a fixed retainer in place by using floss threading device. With proper flossing, there is no reason that fixed retainers, if needed, cannot be left in place indefinitely.

Failure of bondable retainer

Failure rates reported for bonded retainers range from 10.3% to 47.0%.The failure rate amongst bonded retainers was 22.9% and the majority of failures occurred during the third year of observation (Årtun et al (1997). Zachrisson also favours bonding to mandibular canines only but uses a 0.032" stainless steel or 0.030 gold-plated wire which is microetched at each end and claims a failure rate of only 8.4% or 4.2% of bonded sites. Oesterle et al (2001) have shown that optimum bond strength for fixed retainers is achieved with the use of a straight 0.030" stainless steel wire with no terminal bend but a microetched end Zachrisson found significantly lower failure rates with the use of 0.0215-inch Penta One multi-strand wire.

The failure rate is approximately twice as great in the maxilla as the mandible, and this is most likely because of occlusal factors. When placing maxillary retainers, care must be taken to ensure the retainer is free from occlusal trauma to reduce the likelihood of failure. The most common site of failure is at the wire/composite interface. Placements of insufficient adhesive and material loss because of abrasion are implicated in the detachment of the wire from the surface of the composite. The use of increased bulk of composites or materials of greater abrasion resistance may improve the longevity of the retainer.

Rogers and Andrews (2004) have claimed a failure rate of 0.009% for lower 3-3 retainers. They suggest using:

• Maintaining a dry field

• Polishing the lingual surfaces of the lower canines with a finishing bur (other authors have

suggested sandblasting)

• Using loops rather than pads for retention (we prefer no loops and microetching)

• Covering the loops with at least 0.25 mm of composite

• Using a posterior composite filling material as a bonding adhesive

• Using 0.025" diameter wire for the retainer so that the increased flexibility makes it less likely

   those masticatory forces will dislodge the wire

• Contouring the composite carefully

• Only bonding to the canines

Krause Retainer

He used pads that are bonded to the cingulum of anterior teeth.

0.0195 round or 0.016x..022 rectangular braided s.s. wire is used.

Disadvantages

Difficulty in positioning accurately in the mouth.

Difficulty in maintaining oral hygiene, more chances of caries and decalcification.

If used in maxillary arch there are chances of interference with lower incisor.

Axellson and Zachrisson (1992) designed a study to

1. Evaluate the bonding success rates of different types of bonded labial retainers.

2. Study the effects on the gingival tissues and enamel adjacent to such retainers.

3. Determine whether the labial retainers are effective, particularly in preventing the reopening of premolar extraction sites in adults.

58

4. Tabulate patient reactions to different types of labial and lingual retainers, compared with removable plates.

The retainer wire used was .0215" Penta-One five-stranded wire, which was shown in an earlier study of direct-bonded lingual retainers to have optimal properties for stabilizing segments of teeth splinted together, while allowing physiological mobility of the individual units. The most notable side effect was the opening of small spaces distal to the retainer wires in a few patients. In these cases, it is likely that tooth-size discrepancies played a role during settling of the occlusions

The results of this study showed that labially bonded .0215 " wires can were a useful supplement to conventional retention in certain situations, including adult premolar extraction cases and cases involving orthodontic correction of impacted canines. More than 95% of the short labial retainers remained intact over the two-year observation period, and patient acceptance was much better than expected.

The longer retainers, on the other hand, were considerably less successful. A combination of factors such as the patient's age, occlusal interference, and moisture contamination may have been responsible. it was often difficult to place the long mandibular retainers out of occlusion, particularly in young patients with short clinical crowns. When bonding close to the gingival margin, there is an increased risk of seepage of gingival crevicular fluid, which would be detrimental to bond strength.

Sadowsky et al (1994) studied whether long-term fixed retention in the mandibular arch, results in long-term stability of the mandibular anterior teeth. In addition, other changes in the dentition and dentofacial relationships were analyzed.

A sample of 22 previously treated orthodontic cases was studied to evaluate long-term stability. All cases were treated non extraction with fixed edgewise appliances and were without retainers a minimum of 5 years. Data were obtained from study models, although 14 of the 22 cases had longitudinal cephalometric radiographs. The average retention time with a mandibular fixed lingual retainer was 8.4 years. During the post treatment stage all variables showed relapse except for the expanded maxillary canines and premolars. However, the mandibular anterior segment demonstrated relatively good alignment which may be a reflection of prolonged mandibular retention.

Årtun (1984) carried out an investigation to

(1) Test the tendency of different types of bonded retainers to accumulate plaque and calculus and

(2) Find out whether long-term use of bonded retainers caused any damage to the teeth involved. Two test groups of patients— one with 3-3 retainers made of 0.032-inch spiral wire, and the other with 3-3 retainers made of 0.032-inch plain wire— and a reference group of persons without 3-3 retainers were compared. Also, a test group of patients with retainers made of flexible spiral wire (0.0195 inch) bonded lingually to each anterior tooth in the maxilla was compared to a reference group of patients with retention plates in the maxilla. All the persons selected had received routine orthodontic treatment with a

multibonded edgewise light wire technique and had been out of active treatment for 1 to 8 years.

Different indices were used to score accumulation of plaque and calculus, prevalence of caries, and periodontal reactions. The findings indicated that there was no basis on which to claim that retainers made of spiral wire accumulated more plaque and calculus than retainers made of plain wire. The presence of a bonded lingual retainer and the occasional accumulation of plaque and calculus gingival to the retainer wire after long-term use caused no apparent damage to the hard and soft tissues adjacent to the wire.

Alternative means to battle relapse

Igarashi, Mitani, Adachi, and Shinoda (1994) studied whether 4-amino-1-hydroxybutylidene-1, 1-bisphosphonate (AHBuBP), could prevent orthodontic tooth movement or relapse in rats when it was administered systemically and topically. The right and left upper first molars were moved buccally for 3 weeks with a uniform standardized expansion spring under systemic administration of AHBuBP every other day. Histological examination showed that in the experimental animals fewer osteoclasts appeared on the alveolar bone surface, and both bone resorption and root resorption were inhibited. Inhibition of tooth movement was also observed when AHBuBP was applied topically. These results suggest that AHBuBP could be useful in enhancing anchorage or retaining teeth in orthodontic treatment.

Lee et al (2001) investigated the effects of bisphosphonate (BP), an inhibitor of bone resorption, on the remodeling of the rat sagittal suture after rapid expansion. Wistar strain male rats were subject to expansion of their sagittal suture following which Risedronate was administered. In one of the groups bisphosphonate administration was combined with mechanical retention. The results demonstrated that the injection of BP after rapid expansion, if combined with mechanical retention, may produce more secure retention by inhibiting bone resorption, indicating a possibility of employing a pharmaceutical aid to decrease the skeletal relapse after mechanotherapy in clinical orthodontics.

Adachi et al (1994) studied the effect of the topical administration of a bisphosphonate on orthodontic tooth movement in rats. The effect of the drug on the anchorage value as well as the enhancement of retention was studied. They concluded that the topical administration of Risedronate inhibited relapse in a dose dependant manner and also that the topical administration of the drug caused a significant dose dependant reduction of tooth movement upon application of orthodontic force enhancing its anchorage potential.

Conclusion

In summary it can be said that retention is not a separate problem or phase of orthodontics but is and will continue to be a problem to be considered in diagnosis and treatment planning. As Oppenheim so aptly phrased it, "Retention is the most difficult problem in orthodontia; in fact, it is the problem."

Bibliography

1. Clark JD, Kerr WJ, Davis MH. CASES--clinical audit; scenarios for evaluation and study. British Dental Journal 1997; 183:108-111.

2. Reitan K. Clinical and histologic observations on tooth movement during and after orthodontic treatment. American Journal of Orthodontics 1967;53:721-745.

3. Edwards JG. A study of the periodontium during orthodontic rotation of teeth. American Journal of Orthodontics 1968; 54:441-461.

4. Richardson ME, Gormley JS. Lower arch crowding in the third decade. European Journal of Orthodontics 1998; 20:597-607.

5. Sadowsky C, Schneider BJ, BeGole EA, Tahir E. Long-term stability after orthodontic treatment: nonextraction with prolonged retention. American Journal of Orthodontics and Dentofacial Orthodpedics 1994;106:243-249.

6. Edwards JG. A long-term prospective evaluation of the circumferential supracrestal fiberotomy in alleviating orthodontic relapse. American Journal of Orthodontics and Dentofacial Orthopedics 1988; 93:380-387.

7. Proffit WR, Fields HW. Contemporary Orthodontics. 2nd ed. St. Louis: Mosby Year Book, 1992.

8. Nielsen IL. Growth Considerations in Stability of Orthodontic Treatment. In: Nanda R, Burstone CJ, eds. Retention and Stability in Orthodontics. Philadelphia: W.B. Saunders Company, 1993:

9. Zachrisson BU. Orthodontics and Periodontics. In: Lindhe J, Karring T, Lang NP, eds. Clinical Periodontology and Implant Dentistry. 3rd ed. Copenhagen: Munksgaard, 1997:741-793.

10. Sharpe W, Reed B, Subtelny JD, A P. Orthodontic relapse, apical root resorption, and crestal alveolar bone levels. American Journal of Orthodontics and Dentofacial Orthopedics 1987; 91:252-258.

11. Wieslander L. Long-term effect of treatment with the headgear-Herbst appliance in the early mixed dentition. Stability or relapse? American Journal of Orthodontics and Dentofacial Orthopedics 1993; 104:319-329.

12. Kaplan H. The logic of modern retention procedures. American Journal of Orthodontics and Dentofacial Orthopedics 1988; 93:325-340.

13. Joondelph DR, Riedel RA. Retention and Relapse. In: Graber TM, Vanarsdall RL, eds. Orthodontics Current Principles and Techniques. 2nd ed. St. Louis: Mosby - Year Book, 1994:908-950.

14. Sauget E, Covell DA, Boero RP, Lieber WS. Comparison of occlusal contacts with use of Hawley and clear overlay retainers. The Angle Orthodontist 1997; 67:223-230.

15. Bearn DR. Bonded orthodontic retainers: a review. American Journal of Orthodontics and Dentofacial Orthopedics 1995; 108:207-213.

16. Artun J, Urbye KS. The effect of orthodontic treatment on periodontal bone support in patients with advanced loss of marginal periodontium. American Journal of Orthodontics and Dentofacial Orthopedics 1988; 93:143-148.

17. Heier EE, De Smit, A A, Wijgaerts IA, Adriaens PA. Periodontal implications of bonded versus removable retainers. American Journal of Orthodontics and Dentofacial Orthopedics 1997; 112:607-616.

18. Zachrisson BU. Third-generation mandibular bonded lingual 3-3 retainer. Journal of Clinical Orthodontics 1995; 29:39-48.

19. Little RM, Riedel RA, Artun J. An evaluation of changes in mandibular anterior alignment from 10 to 20 years post-retention. American Journal of Orthodontics and Dentofacial Orthopedics 1988; 93:423-428.

20. Little RM. Stability and relapse of dental arch alignment. British Journal of Orthodontics 1990; 17:235-241.

21. Richardson ME. Late lower arch crowding facial growth or forward drift? European Journal of Orthodontics 1979; 1:219-225.

22. Richardson ME. Lower incisor corwding in the young adult. American Journal of Orthodontics and Dentofacial Orthopedics 1992;101:132-137.

23. Surbeck BT, Artun J, Hawkins NR, Leroux B. Associations between initial, posttreatment, and post-retention alignment of maxillary anterior teeth. American Journal of Orthodontics and Dentofacial Orthopedics 1998; 113:186-195.

24. Mills JRE. The stability of the lower labial segment. Transactions of the British Society for the Study of Orthodontics 1967; 54:11-24.

25. Schulhof RJ, Allen RW, Walters RD, Dreskin M. The mandibular dental arch: Part I, lower incisor position. The Angle Orthodontist 1977; 47:280-287.

26. Mills JRE. The stability of the lower labial segment. A cephalometric survey. Dent Pract Dent Rec 1968; 18:293-306.

27. Houston WJ, Edler R. Long-term stability of the lower labial segment relative to the A-Pog line. British Journal of Orthodontics 1990; 12:302-310.

28. Lopez-Gavito G, Wallen TR, Little RM, Joondeph DR. Anterior open-bite malocclusion: a longitudinal 10-year post-retention evaluation of orthodontically treated patients. American Journal of Orthodontics and Dentofacial Orthopedics 1985; 87:175-186.

29. Harris EF, Vaden JL, Dunn KL, Behrents RG. Effects of patient age on post-orthodontic stability in Class II, division 1 malocclusions. American Journal of Orthodontics 1994; 105:25-34.

30. Harris EF, Vaden JL. Posttreatment stability in adult and adolescent orthodontic patients: a cast analysis. International Journal of Adult Orthodontics and Orthognathic Surgery 1994; 9:19-29.

31. Årtun J, Spadafora A and Shapiro P. A 3-year follow-up of various types of orthodontic canine-to-canine retainers. European Journal of Orthodontics1997; 19: 501-509.

32. Zachrisson BU. Important aspects of long-term stability. Journal of Clinical Orthodontics1997; 31: 562-583.

33. Oesterle LJ, Shellhart WC and Henderson S. Enhancing wire-composite bond strength of bonded retainers with wire surface treatment. American Journal of Orthodontics and Dentofacial Orthopaedics 2001; 119:625-631.

34. Christopher k. kesling. Permanent Retainer Activation with the Self-Activated Loop System. J. Clin. Orthod. 2002:413-415.

35. Aldo macchi, Nunzio cirulli. Fixed Active Retainer for Minor Anterior Tooth Movement. J. Clin. Orthod. 2000: 48-50.

36. Miyawaki, S.; Yasuhara, M.; and Koh, Y.: Discomfort caused by bonded lingual orthodontic appliances in adult patients examined by retrospective questionnaire. Am. J. Orthod Dentofac Orthop; 115:83-88, 1999.

37. Rogers MB and Andrews II LJ. A dependable technique for bonding a 3 x 3 retainer. Am. J. Orthod Dentofac Orthop 2004;126: 231-233

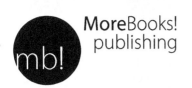
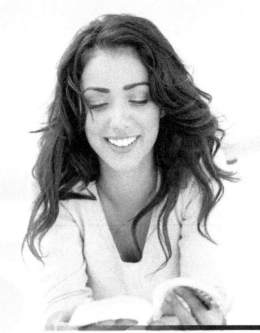